BEDROOM SECRETS FOR MEN

HOW TO SATISFY YOUR WOMAN IN THE BEDROOM

ANTHONY EKANEM

Made with ♥ on the Notion Press Platform
www.notionpress.com

Contents

Preface

The need to write this report arose because I wanted to help married men and women enjoy intimacy with their spouses. One of the most common reasons why marriages fail these days is the lack of sexual satisfaction by either of the spouses.

Experts say sex is very key to maintaining successful marital relationships. There are so many benefits to being intimate in your marital relationship. Interestingly, there are health and emotional benefits attached to sex. With these in mind, being intimate with your spouse should not just be for the sake of sex but should be because of the health and emotional benefits as well as the intimacy it brings into your relationship.

Highlighted below are some of the importance of sex in a marital relationship. This is not exhaustive. Let us start with the emotional benefits of sex.

The Emotional Benefits of Sex

1. It creates intimacy in a relationship.
2. It makes partners emotionally closer.
3. It deepens the connection between partners.
4. It is used to make up after a disagreement.
5. It is used for gratification.
6. Sex assures partners that they want and need each other.

The Physical/Health Benefits of Sex

1. It boosts self-esteem.
2. It boosts the immune system.

3. It helps burn calories (one of the best ways to watch your weight!)
4. Having regular sex helps in stress relief.
5. It reduces blood pressure.
6. For stronger pelvic floor muscles.
7. For better sleep.
8. It improves heart health.
9. It helps with pain.
10. More ejaculations may make prostate cancer less likely.

For you to have a healthy relationship, sex must be a part of that relationship. Sex can help a relationship get better. According to experts, once sex is taken out of a relationship, issues like poor communication, the most dangerous problem couples with poor sex life encounter, lack of trust, betrayals, poor libido and many more, set in.

Endeavour to spice up your relationship with quality sex to live healthy emotionally and physically. But know that Testosterone is the most important male sex hormone. In males, it is mainly responsible for the development of the sex organs, the formation and maintenance of typical male sexual characteristics, sperm production, and the control of male desire. Supplying the body with enough Vitamin D has positive effects on testosterone levels.

CHAPTER ONE

How To Have Sex

Having sex can sometimes mean many different sexual activities, but usually, it means sexual intercourse. The most common definition of sexual intercourse is an act that involves a man putting his erect penis inside a woman's vagina.

Foreplay, and getting sexually excited.

Sexual intercourse between a man and a woman usually starts with both getting sexually excited. This is sometimes referred to as foreplay and might involve sexual activities such as kissing, cuddling, and touching each other. Foreplay is important as it means a woman's vagina begins to get moist and a man gets an erection. If the woman's vagina does not get moist enough, then having sexual intercourse could be difficult or painful for the woman (and/or the man).

Protection during sex

If two people have sex and one of them has a sexually transmitted disease (STD) then they could pass it on to the other person. Using a condom is the best way to prevent any infection from being passed from one person to the other. If a man and woman are having sexual intercourse and using a condom for protection against pregnancy or infections, they should put it on the man's penis as soon as he gets an erection. Some men say they worry about using condoms in case they lose their erection or have difficulty putting the condom on. You could get some condoms and practice beforehand. Condoms come with instructions in words and pictures which show exactly how to use them.

After the condom is on, the man or woman can guide his penis into the vagina. The couple then move their bodies so that his penis moves up and down inside her vagina. This usually rubs the penis and makes the man sexually excited so that he has an orgasm. The movement might also rub the woman's clitoris (or sensitive areas inside her vagina) so she can have an orgasm. But this often takes practice and a bit of experimentation to get it right!

Does having sex hurt?

Having sex does not usually hurt, though first-time sex may be a bit uncomfortable for a woman because her hymen (a thin layer of skin that partially covers the entrance to the vagina) may be stretched or torn. Some girls are born without a hymen and some tear theirs when inserting tampons or during sports. A torn hymen may cause a little bleeding, but it does not usually last long. Sex is not usually painful for a man.

The best way to ensure pain-free sex is for both partners to *relax* and take their time. After the first time, sex should become more comfortable. The vagina is very stretchy and will usually accommodate a penis (even a large one) with ease. However, a woman may experience pain when having sexual intercourse if her vagina does not produce enough natural lubrication. Extra vaginal fluids are usually produced when a woman becomes sexually excited to allow the penis to enter the vagina easily. If a woman is tense or rushing when she has sex, her vagina may not become moist enough to allow the penis to move in and out smoothly. Stress can also cause the muscles in the vagina to involuntarily tense up, making penetration difficult and painful. The best way to ensure pain-free sex is for both partners to relax and take their time.

Extra lubrication might also help and can be bought from many chemists and supermarkets. When using a condom, a water-based lubricant (like KY jelly) must be used, as oil-based lubricants like Vaseline can cause the condom to disintegrate.

Which position is best for having sex?

There are quite a lot of different positions for sexual intercourse. One of the most common is the *missionary position*, where a woman lies on her back and a man lies on top of her. A man and woman might also lie on their sides, the woman may sit on top of the man, or she may kneel on all fours while the man puts his penis into her vagina from behind. If couples are in a position where the woman's clitoris is not being stimulated, they can do this with their fingers.

What does sex feel like?

Sexual activities such as kissing are important too. Similar things happen to most people's bodies when they have sex - they get sensitive and warm and excited and may have an orgasm. Enjoying sexual activities with another person is possible whether you have an orgasm or not. Not being able to have an orgasm with another person doesn't mean that you don't fancy them or love them. Your emotions might be different each time you have a sexual experience, depending on the circumstances. Having sex can be one of the most intense and pleasurable physical and emotional experiences a person can have.

How do you have an orgasm?

When sexual excitement builds up and reaches a peak, a person might experience an orgasm, also called a climax, or 'coming'. The sexual excitement might start from someone masturbating on their own, or through kissing, masturbating, or having sex with another person.

Sexual excitement usually grows gradually, and a person feels more and more pleasure and a kind of exciting tension. All the feelings of tension then disappear when the orgasm happens, and the person experiences feelings of intense pleasure. The feeling can be so strong that a person might not be able to see or hear or think about anything for a moment. They might even groan and call out with pleasure. Orgasms usually last only a few seconds but the feelings might last a lot longer.

When a man has an orgasm, he ejaculates. This means that sperm mixed with semen comes out of the end of his penis in a sticky white fluid. After a man has ejaculated, he loses his erection and usually needs to stop for a while. When a woman has an orgasm, her vagina often becomes very wet, but she can continue being sexually aroused as long as she likes. Some women can experience more than one orgasm without stopping.

If a person doesn't have an orgasm, it doesn't mean anything is wrong. Worrying about reaching an orgasm or being nervous is quite likely to make it hard for a person to relax enough to have one.

How long does sex last?

It depends on what you mean by sex! The time people devote to doing sexual things can last from a few minutes to several hours or even a whole day! The actual act of sexual intercourse will often last until a man has an orgasm (ejaculates or comes), although there's nothing wrong with stopping before this point.

A man might find he comes very quickly the first time he has sexual intercourse. Usually, sexual intercourse lasts longer as people get more experienced and know what to expect. But with a new partner, it can take time for people to get used to each other. Sex will usually be different every time - it depends on how couples feel and what they want.

Is sex noisy?

Only if you want it to be! Some people do make noises when they have sex. They might moan or groan with pleasure or even cry out. Some people talk to each other. Others don't speak or make any noise. But your body might make noises that you can't help - squelching and squishing. These might be embarrassing or funny, but they are perfectly normal.

How often do people have sex?

Sexual activities differ from couple to couple. Sexual appetite is entirely a matter of personal taste. Some people have sex once or twice a day and others once a month. It probably varies for most people depending on whether they are in a relationship, how busy they are and how they feel. Most people think about sex far more often than they do it.

How do you have oral sex?

Oral sex is when one person licks or sucks another person's penis or vagina. When oral sex is done to a man it is sometimes called a *blow job*. When it is done to a woman it is sometimes called *licking out*. If two people have oral sex with each other at the same time it is sometimes called a "*69*" because of the shape their bodies make. A woman cannot get pregnant by giving oral sex to a man, even if she swallows his sperm.

Oral sex can be a very intense and intimate experience. Some people enjoy giving oral sex or having it. Other people feel uncomfortable about the idea and don't want to do it. Sometimes people feel pressure to have oral sex when they don't want to. It is very important to think about what the other person wants if you want to have oral sex. Some sexually transmitted infections can be passed on through oral sex.

How do you masturbate?

A woman usually masturbates by rubbing, stroking, or squeezing her clitoris. The clitoris is the most sensitive sexual part of a woman. She might also touch her breasts and other sensitive areas of her body. A man usually masturbates by stroking, rubbing, or 'pumping' his penis, and may concentrate particularly on the tip, which is the most sensitive part. Masturbation is sometimes referred to as *playing with yourself*, or, especially with men, *jerking off, a hand job, or wanking.*

There is no physical reason why you should or shouldn't masturbate. It is not true that you'll go blind if you masturbate or that you will become weak or lose your health. People don't necessarily begin masturbating when they reach puberty. Some people hardly ever masturbate, and others masturbate a lot. It varies according to how a person feels. Many people masturbate even when they are in a relationship with someone. Masturbation can last as long as you want, but generally, people masturbate for between a few minutes and half an hour.

It is not possible to masturbate too much, though you should stop if you start to make yourself feel sore. Some people think that if a man doesn't masturbate his testes will fill up with sperm. This is not true; the sperm are just absorbed into his body. It is also not true that women who think about sex or masturbate are 'easy'.

Things You Should Never Do While Having Sex

When you are in bed with your lover, the last thing you want to do is turn them off. That said, here are a few common blunders that you should not commit.

1. Not kissing

Believe it or not, many people (and this includes women) don't kiss their partner when they're having sex. Why? Perhaps because the positioning doesn't allow for it or they are too eager to climax and feel that it might break the rhythm. Nevertheless, it is highly recommended that you try to kiss your partner during the act - it will only add to the experience.

2. Biting before your partner is ready

While many people enjoy an aggressive partner, biting any part of their body before they are aroused may lead to pain and discomfort (and might even lessen the chances of any further action) or simply scare them off. So, make sure your partner is fully excited before you bite their ear, shoulders, neck or any other part of their body.

3. Ignoring everything but sexualized parts

Genitals are great, no doubt, but you should pay attention to other parts of your lover's body and focus for some time on their entire body - knees, wrists, back and stomach are highly erogenous zones for men as well as women. Gently caressing these areas will help excite your partner further; in turn, increasing the chances of their pleasuring you back.

4. Putting your weight on your partner

It is okay to lose yourself in the moment every once in a while and go crazy on your lover. But when you are lying on top of them, you must be careful not to drop your weight on them. Chocking them or hindering their ability to breathe will anyway kill the moment and any chances of some good action.

5. Climaxing too soon/too late

You need to have good control over your muscles to ensure that you can ejaculate at an appropriate time. Too soon and you may leave your partner unsatisfied; too late and it might leave your partner feeling as if they are pumping iron at the gym. To avoid this, spend a lot more time on *foreplay* (this will help men as well as women). If you take too long and can only ejaculate via manual stimulation, do your best to get your partner to orgasm and then they can return the favour.

6. Not warning your partner before you climax

If you are going to let go - and this applies even to women - whether during oral sex or intercourse, you need to tell your partner beforehand. Something as simple as "I'm going to let go," will suffice. Your partner deserves to know.

7. Treating sex like porn

Although some couples enjoy having raunchy sex, you would be wise to talk to your partner before you engage in such behaviour. If you begin being nasty with your lover without knowing if they like it first, chances are the scenario won't end on a happy note.

8. Staying quiet

Do you like to hear it when your partner is having a good time? So pay them the same respect and speak up when you are enjoying yourself. Something as simple as a little moan, or even saying something like, "that feels so good," will encourage them and educate them further on your moan zones.

9. Mechanical act

It may feel comfortable for you to pump away as you do at the gym, but you will quickly discover that most people don't enjoy such an act. Mix it up a little bit; go fast at times, then slowly. Be creative and you'll find yourself enjoying some variation too.

Mistakes Men Make in Bed – And How to Avoid Them

When it comes to what women want in bed, men tend to make serious avoidable mistakes like these –

A recent survey suggests that most men are not the skillful lovers they think themselves to be. When it comes to the fundamentals, men tend to make some serious mistakes in the sack. Here are the avoidable ones.

1. Silent play

No matter the circumstances, most men tend to be eerily silent during the entire act. You may think that's fine, but this makes your woman feel alienated. It makes her wonder if she's pleasuring you. There's no need to exaggerate your feelings, but you can let your partner know you are genuinely enjoying her company. The occasional moans and groans are not such a bad thing.

2. Foreplay is not a means to an end

Most men tend to breeze through it - the effortless kissing here, and caressing there, as they undress. But in too much anticipation of a great act, you may appear desperate to begin. And that won't score you any brownie points in the long run. Take it slowly. Enjoy every aspect of the encounter as you get to know the woman you are with. Women enjoy a well-paced build-up - the making-out, the undressing, the reciprocal oral sex. This will also lead to a more fulfilling encounter; and perhaps, a standing invitation for more.

3. Forget the big "O"

Besides, when you approach sex with a clear focus on only reaching an orgasm, you may lose sight of the path to the climactic moment. Don't pressure yourself, or your partner, to hit the finish line as quickly as possible. Rather than rush it, why not enjoy the experience as a whole? You'll prolong your pleasure, and your partner will feel like she's with a man who knows what he's doing. The conclusion, though delayed, will be a lot more satisfying for both.

4. The fingers carefully

Although digital penetration is considered a normal part of foreplay, some men get over-eager and, confuse their fingers for penises. As a result, they finger their partners with a vigour reserved for sex. This also reflects that they have no clue what a woman wants, which is why they have resolved to go hard and fast. Instead, you should aim for a more measured approach; make her get used to the feel of your fingers as you gradually insert more of them.

5. Sensitize Yourself to her wants

If you think that simply pounding away at a woman during sex is a major turn-on, you are wrong. Yet, many men are convinced that it will ultimately bring their partners to orgasm. But women are sensitive souls. They appreciate nuance, feeling and deep emotion. So, rather than thrusting away from beginning to end, you'll want to vary your speed throughout sex. Gauge your partner's response, take it as a lead and simply go with the flow. If she asks you to go harder, oblige. But if the moment calls for it, go slowly. The key is to sensitize yourself to what she wants, and not what you want.

6. Go easy with the clitoris

Women enjoy clitoral stimulation more than any sort of penetration. So never ignore her clitoris. Yet, at the same time, don't treat it like a scratch card and rub it relentlessly to make your partner climax. Remember, the clitoris is extremely sensitive, so too much force can prove painful.

7. Keep her entire body in mind

When you have sex, you aim to please the woman you are with. So it makes sense that many men focus on the one or two sensitive areas of her body like the neck or thighs. However, the next step is not to look for other ways to please her. Though this notion is understandable, it is also incredibly short-sighted. The law of diminishing returns applies everywhere — even in the bedroom. If you've worked her neck for a while, move down to her breasts. And you may not want to focus heavily on her clitoris. Overstimulation can sometimes prove unpleasant. So, keep things varied. As the age-old adage goes, variety is the spice of life.

8. Rough now, but be sweet later

There's nothing wrong with a little roughness if it's consensual. But you should never take it too far (no one wants to leave the bedroom in need of medical attention) and you should always remember to show some compassion afterwards. When it's all over, make sure you pay attention to her immediate needs, which will likely mean some snuggling and cuddling.

9. Don't stress about the G-Spot

The location of the G-Spot (Grafenberg Spot) has long eluded men. It is widely understood to be a couple of inches up the anterior vaginal wall, between the vaginal opening and the urethra. Your search will probably be less scientific, once you've inserted your fingers into her vagina, and curled them as though you were asking someone to come toward you; the spot you're looking for will feel rippled. But don't let that elusive area become the be-all, end-all of your sex life.

CHAPTER TWO

Pre-Mature Ejaculation

First, pat yourself on the back for having the desire to gather the information that can cure your premature ejaculation (PE). The sooner you recognize you have this problem, the faster and easier it is to fully cure it.

If you were like me, then a night of lovemaking was a cause for nervousness, anxiety, and embarrassment. I thought of every excuse why I couldn't last more than 30 seconds and promised I would last longer next time, only for my partner to get more frustrated and me more ashamed.

The good news is that PE is one of the easiest male sexual dysfunctions to cure and there is no need for long-term medical treatment.

How does ejaculation occur?

Ejaculation, controlled by the central nervous system, happens when friction on the genitalia and other forms of sexual stimulation provide impulses that are sent up the spinal cord and into the brain.

Ejaculation has two phases:

Phase I - emission

The tubes that store and transport sperm from the testes contract to squeeze the sperm toward the base of the penis through the prostate gland and into the urethra. The seminal vesicles release secretions that combine with the sperm to make semen. Ejaculation is unstoppable at this stage.

Phase II - ejaculation

The muscles at the base of the penis and urethra contract, forcing semen out of the penis (ejaculation and orgasm) while the bladder neck contracts. Orgasm can occur without the delivery of semen (ejaculation) from the penis; this causes a "dry" orgasm. Normally, erections decline following ejaculation.

What is Premature Ejaculation?

Premature ejaculation is uncontrolled ejaculation either before or shortly after sexual penetration, with minimal sexual stimulation and before the person wishes. It may result in an unsatisfactory sexual experience for both partners. This can increase the anxiety that may contribute to the problem. Premature ejaculation is one of the most common forms of male sexual dysfunction and has probably affected every man at some point in their life.

It is one of the most common male sexual disorders, affecting about 20-30% of men of all ages. Premature ejaculation is a frustrating problem that can reduce the enjoyment of sex, harm relationships and impair quality of life.

What causes premature ejaculation?

Most cases of premature ejaculation do not have a clear cause. With sexual experience and age, men often learn to delay orgasm. Premature ejaculation may occur with a new partner, only in certain sexual situations, or if it has been a long time since the last ejaculation. Psychological factors such as anxiety, guilt, or depression can cause premature ejaculation. In some cases, premature ejaculation may be related to a medical cause such as hormonal problems, injury, or a side effect of certain medicines.

Excess stress and anxiety can be enough to cause PE in men. Becoming nervous and tense right before intercourse will always make the situation worse. Also, men may become over mentally stimulated, especially if they are new to having sex.

Almost all cases of PE can be traced back to genetics, sensitivity and intensity, poor masturbation habits, or lack of understanding of the ejaculatory process. Some men's bodies are simply wired to ejaculate faster. This is because of the way they were born, or that they have programmed themselves through poor masturbation habits. Also, some men just can't help but organism faster because the stimulation is just too intense to handle.

Can Premature Ejaculation develop later in life?

Premature ejaculation can occur at any age. Surprisingly, ageing appears not to be a cause of premature ejaculation. However, the ageing process typically causes changes in erectile function and ejaculation. Erections may not be as firm or as large. Erections may be maintained for a shorter period before ejaculating. The feeling that an ejaculation is about to happen may be shorter. These factors can result in an older man having an ejaculation earlier than when he was younger.

Premature ejaculation, although very curable, affects each man differently. What may work for some men may not work for others. In other words, there is no one solution for curing every man's PE. Therefore, approach the following information like a road map which will show you the direction you need to take to cure your premature ejaculation.

What are the symptoms?

The main symptom of premature ejaculation is uncontrolled ejaculation either before or shortly after intercourse begins. Ejaculation occurs before the person wishes it, with minimal sexual stimulation.

If you are not sure you classify as having PE, here are some facts you can go by.

1. You routinely finish before you and your partner would like to.
2. Your inability to last long enough is causing your partner distress.
3. You typically finish within two minutes of intercourse.

If you find you have at least one of these traits, chances are that you are suffering from premature ejaculation.

Fixing premature ejaculation is very possible and most men can be fully cured. To start treating your PE, here is what NOT to do.

1. The first is to fall into the wrong mindset.

Don't let the negative feelings of having PE get to you. It is important to realize that this condition is not your fault. You need to explain and be honest with your partner that you are not doing this on purpose and that you want to seek out a real solution. Communication between partners is key if you are trying to come up with a solution.

2. Don't Do the Wrong Things

One of the first and easiest things you can do is to relax and avoid stress. Stress is the enemy as far as PE goes. Stress is bad whether it relates to your performance in bed or at work. Also, you do not want to lose emotional control. Being angry or emotionally charged right before sex can cause you to lose control within a few minutes.

When trying to cure PE, a lot of men go for applicators like numbing creams or sprays. This is the most common solution men use to try to treat their PE. Although these may offer a very temporary solution, they are not recommended if you are trying to fix your PE for good. One of the first things you need to do when trying to last longer in bed is to be aware of sensations and feelings in your body and recognize your arousal level. Numbing creams often cause men to go limp and usually lower the sensation you and your partner experience during sex. Also, do you want to run to the bathroom to apply a spray each time before sex? I didn't think so.

Like numbing creams, it is also important to avoid herbal pills and other medications designed to delay ejaculation. Often, herbal pills will not do much to lessen the intensity men feel. Herbal pills, even if they do work, are not permanent solutions. You will have to continue taking these for the rest of your life before having intercourse.

Also, some therapists recommend taking anti-depressant-type drugs. These drugs have had success delaying ejaculation but often come with several side effects, some serious. Sometimes these types of drugs can result in loss of libido or extreme difficulty in ejaculating. For them to work, you must take them before having sex regularly for the rest of your life.

Natural Cure for Pre-Mature Ejaculation

The good news is that premature ejaculation can be cured naturally and permanently without the need to use any expensive and often very dangerous PE drugs. To do this, you have to read the remaining part of this report very carefully and APPLY the techniques mentioned therein.

1. Control Your Arousal

One of the first things you can do to end your PE is to manage your arousal control. Arousal is the sensations you go through when you become stimulated. To be able to last longer, you have to understand exactly how stimulated you are and how close you are to reach what therapists call '*the point of no return*' or when the nervous system automatically takes over the ejaculatory processes. By better understanding just how aroused you are, you can better position yourself to control how long you will last and when to lessen arousal and stimulation.

The arousal process goes through ten levels.

Level 1: This is when you are soft, with no erection.

Level 2: You are beginning to feel aroused but just a little.

Level 3: Your penis is getting erect but not that hard – maybe because you have seen her breasts or buttocks.

Level 4: Your penis is now hard ...but not VERY hard.

Level 5: At this stage, you are VERY hard and ready to penetrate her.

Level 6: You are already inside her and your arousal level is starting to go up speedily

Level 7/8: At this stage, you are highly aroused. You are enjoying the sex but you can still control yourself.

Level 9: You can feel highly aroused and you can feel that you are about to ejaculate but you can still hold it.

Level 10: You are about to ejaculate and you cannot control yourself. Even if the sky is going to fall on you, you will still ejaculate. This is the "*point of no return*".

If you feel close to 8 or 9, then stop thrusting, and let yourself unwind back down to level 5. Once you are not as aroused, then you can proceed again. Use the time you are unwinding to do something different during your lovemaking. This will not only help you last longer but make the love-making session more interesting for her.

A woman needs attention to all parts of her body to feel fulfilled. Focus on teasing her with words and pressing sensuous areas and hot buttons all over her body. Also, make sure to alternate between deep and shallow thrusting. Deep thrusting will present less friction on the glands.

2. Use the Right Position

One of the easiest ways to last longer, especially if you are too sensitive, is to use a position that puts less pressure on the sensitive areas of your penis.

If there is direct stimulation on the glands of the head, your chances of lasting long will be cut significantly. Try to spread her legs apart during intercourse and thrust more deeply pressing your pelvic area against her. Make sure to avoid the missionary position. Although this is the most used, this is the worst for men trying to last longer. Also, try a position in which she is on top. Not only will this be more stimulating for her but it will help you last longer, too.

3. Developing the PC Muscle

All men have a PC muscle located between the anus and testes. This contracts involuntarily before ejaculation. To prevent involuntary contractions from happening, these muscles must be developed and controlled. There are various exercises you can do to strengthen your PC muscles to stop ejaculation. Basic exercising involves contracting the PC muscle for many seconds and then relaxing it. Most men who have PE can barely hold this for a few seconds. Once you gain control of the PC muscle, you can relax and contract during intercourse to help prolong ejaculation.

4. Breathing Techniques

Have you ever focused on how you breathe during intercourse? Most men breathe very rapidly taking short shallow breaths. For men suffering from PE, this is the worst way to breathe. Instead, focus on diaphragmatic breathing and taking long, deep, and relaxing breaths. When you feel yourself becoming overstimulated, inhale for a count of five then exhale for five. This will calm your nerves and allow you to last much longer. When breathing, make sure only the stomach moves up and down. Most men make the mistake of breathing too shallowly.

How to Last Longer in Bed

Whether you regularly experience premature ejaculation, a common sexual problem among men, or simply want to find ways to make sex last longer, there are plenty of things you can do both during and before sex to prevent yourself from getting too excited too quickly. Read on.

Before sex

1. Relax and be positive. Premature ejaculation is as much a physical issue as a mental one. Try not to create a self-fulfilling prophecy by labelling yourself as sexually incompetent in any way. Approaching sex with confidence, self-respect, and a positive attitude rather than fear and self-doubt can make all the difference for both you and your partner.

2. "Practice" with yourself. Masturbation is perfectly healthy and natural, and doing it regularly can help you build up your stamina, prevent premature ejaculation, and even relieve stress and anxiety. Plus, the more time you spend with yourself, the more familiar you will become with your body so that you can more easily recognize when you get too excited. That way, during sex, you can know when to slow down or change positions before it's too late.

3. Find a regular sexual partner (if possible). Men tend to get particularly worked up during their first time with a new woman, especially if this woman is somebody he has been lusting after for a long time. Realize that sometimes it isn't *you*, but rather, how attracted to and excited you are about being in bed with *her*. And that's perfectly ok. Being in a monogamous relationship is a great way to improve your performance in bed, and the more time you spend with one person, the more comfortable and confident you will feel during sex.

4. Cut down on alcohol, tobacco, and other drugs. Using these substances in excess may interfere with your ability to control ejaculation.

During sex

1. Don't skip foreplay. Studies have shown that couples that indulge in foreplay report having sex for longer than those who don't. Instead of getting right down to business, take some time to cuddle, kiss, and touch one another, and so on. The more time you spend on foreplay, the longer you'll be in bed together. If you get too excited during foreplay, stop her from doing whatever she's doing and focus all your attention on her instead.

2. Change positions often. This can shift your attention. Plus, exploring different sexual positions can make sex more exciting and ensure that both partners are satisfied. Also, don't be afraid to stop having sex temporarily to focus on her.

3. Let her be in control. The person who is in control is usually the one experiencing most of the pleasure; letting her be in control can help decrease some of the sensitivity you feel.

4. Try to distract yourself. If you find yourself getting too excited during sex, try to distract yourself from how turned on you are by thinking about something completely unrelated to the situation, like work or school. Temporarily diverting your attention can help you relax and slow down.

Whatever you think of, make sure that it's something that doesn't turn you on sexually in any way.

5. Take slow, deep breaths. Many men find that breathing slowly and deeply during sex can help them last longer. This can be attributed to the fact that breathing helps us relax. Try to breathe deep into your belly. Feel it expanding as you inhale. It may also help to hold your breath for two or three seconds before exhaling, slowly. This holding can have a calming effect.

6. Get Out of Your Head. Performance anxiety is the number one killer of sustaining an erection. Shift your thinking to a more confident inner voice, as opposed to a worried voice. When you begin to feel anxiety, the strategy is to stop, take a breath, and then focus on how things feel in the body. Stay out of your *head* and get into your *body*—focus on the feelings that your body is producing for you.

7. Change things up. The best thing to do if you're getting close to the edge? Take your penis out and rub just the head of it sensually up and down and between her labia. Vaginas have lots of nerve endings clustered in the lower portion of their vaginal canal, so this move will still be very enjoyable for her to experience.

8. Slow down! Instead of the fast-paced jackhammering style that many men are so fond of, try taking your time. Sex at a slower pace leads to a more connected experience for both people. It's more sensual because you are caressing and exploring the rest of her body. Kiss her neck, nuzzle her ear, and let your hands gently explore her body. The most important thing to keep in mind that will help you last longer? Enjoy the *journey* that leads to your destination.

9. Exercise your PC muscle. PC muscles (or pubococcygeus muscles) are the ones that stretch from the anus to the urinary sphincter. To figure out how to squeeze and contract the PC muscles, try stopping your urine flow while you're in the middle of peeing. You'll know it when you try it. Daily PC muscle exercises will help you to pump yourself up. Squeezing those muscles triggers good blood flow to the penis, which in turn leads to mental confidence.

Other Tips on Lasting Longer in Bed

Think for a second about what causes you to orgasm. I mean, you don't ever just orgasm out of nowhere, do you? There must be something to cause you to orgasm. And what causes you to orgasm is the pleasure or stimulation, you experience. Now, the problem that you have, if you're not lasting long enough, is that you are allowing yourself to experience pleasure, or stimulation, at a high intensity. This high intensity of stimulation is what causes you to orgasm earlier than you want. When you get this, understanding the real cause of premature ejaculation is simple.

You + Uncontrolled Intense Stimulation = Premature Ejaculation

The question is how can you use this knowledge to get you to last longer in bed?

And the answer is simple. To last longer in bed all you need to do is take control of your stimulation. Because if you can take control of your stimulation and reduce it, then naturally it will take longer for you to orgasm. But this is something that most men just never do. Most men just assume that there's nothing they can do. They assume they must just be unlucky, it's their wife, girlfriend, or partner's fault, they were born with the wrong "gene", they're too old, too young, have the wrong penis size, etc.

The truth is that if you're not lasting as long as you want to in bed, then all you need to do is take control of

your stimulation. When you realize that what you are doing before and during sex is affecting how long you last suddenly you can start to dramatically influence how long you last. When you start acknowledging that every little action you take before and during sex is having some kind of impact on your stimulation, then it becomes easy to make a change. It becomes easy to see how doing x, y or z is causing you to be overstimulated and therefore is making you orgasm. So, the bottom line of what I'm trying to get through is that you are in control.

The things you do before and during sex have a very real impact on how you last. It's not your age, penis size, genes or how you were born; it's the actions you take.

And this is great news because this puts you in the driver's seat. And the next five steps will tell you exactly which actions to take before and during sex to reduce your stimulation and therefore last significantly longer than you ever thought was possible.

The positions you use during sex can have a dramatic effect on how long you last in bed.

So in this step, I want to show which positions can help you last significantly longer in bed and which positions can hugely reduce how long you last. So when it comes to positions, ***lasting longer is as simple as using positions that cause you less stimulation more often than the positions that cause you a lot of stimulation.***

1. Low stimulation positions

These are the positions you'll want to favour more often when having sex. One great low-stimulation position is **standing up**. This can involve you carrying your woman or just having sex in a position that involves you standing up. The reason this works so well is that when you're standing up, tension and pressure are directed away from your penis.

When you're standing up, energy is being spent in your legs keeping you standing and if you're carrying or holding her then energy is also being spent in your upper body. Since energy is needed elsewhere besides your penis, this takes the pressure off, reduces the stimulation experienced by your penis and therefore makes lasting longer easier.

Another great low-stimulation position is having **her on top** while you lie down. Now I know a lot of men struggle with this position because they feel like they've got no control, but the fact is they're just not using the position correctly. When you're in this position there are two ways you can reduce your stimulation very effectively. Firstly, you can take control by grabbing her hips. By holding her hips, you communicate to her that you're in charge and therefore you control her thrusting speed. If you want to slow her down, you can by making it obvious by the way you hold her.

Secondly, this position is unlike most other positions where you must make some kind of movement for them to work. This means that in this position you can fully relax your body. Most men when they get in this position forget about stimulation control, get overwhelmed and orgasm quickly. But when you're in this position take the time to relax. Take some slow, deep breaths and consciously relax all your muscles. Allow all the muscles in your legs to relax. By relaxing your muscles, you reduce the tension in your body. And with less tension in your body, you reduce your stimulation and make it more difficult for your body to orgasm. So, if you combine these two benefits this position works great.

2. High stimulation positions

This varies from man to man, but often the missionary position (where the woman lies down facing up, with the man on top facing down) is very stimulating. Because no tension is getting diverted away like in a standing-up position and it's much harder to relax like when you, the man, are on the bottom, this position can quite easily cause premature ejaculation. The problem with this position is that it's just so stimulating to the man. If you can reduce your time spent in this position or find variations of it that don't cause you to feel as much stimulation then I highly recommend doing that.

3. Using position changes

In changing positions you often get a quick break from sex, even if it's just for 10 seconds or so. This 10-second or more break can be very valuable, especially if you're getting close to orgasm because taking a quick break can sometimes "reset" your stimulation so you'll have a few more minutes before orgasm.

In the future, look to use your position changes tactically when you're close to orgasm to help you last longer. Here I want to give you a thrusting technique that is literally "plug-and-play". By this I mean you don't need to think about it, work on it, practice it, or anything like that. This one is as simple as doing it. And when you do it right, you can add several minutes to how long you last, while giving her some great pleasure at the same time. Now I call this thrusting technique the "Full Thrust" stimulation reducer.

And how it works is like this...

When having sex most men will thrust in and out fully. They'll go in as deep as they can, and they'll withdraw almost out. The problem with this thrusting style is that it is highly stimulating. And as you learned above, you want to do everything you can to reduce your overall stimulation to a controllable level so you can last longer. But at the same time, you don't want to thrust in such a way that it doesn't give her pleasure in any way.

Now, before I tell you the technique, you need to understand this ...

The mushroom-like end of your penis (also known as the "Glans") is the most sensitive part of your penis. And since it's the most sensitive, this means it causes you to experience the most amount of stimulation and pleasure. So, if you can reduce how much stimulation your glans receive, then you can last much longer. In the "Full Thrust" stimulation reducer you aim to thrust and pleasure your woman, while at the same time minimizing the stimulation to your glans.

The way to do this is as follows.

When you thrust, go in as deep as you can without hurting her. And once you're this deep continue to thrust, but only withdraw an inch or two. So while you're thrusting, all the time you're still staying very deep inside her. What this means is that your glans stay deep inside her as well. And this means your glans don't get close to the entrance of her vagina, which happens to be the tightest and most stimulation-causing part of the vagina.

So by keeping your glans well away from the entrance to her vagina, it gets very little stimulation, but at the same time, she will notice virtually no difference, because she's still experiencing plenty of thrusting. So while you're reducing your stimulation massively, she's still getting pleasured as much as normal. In a nutshell, you last longer, while she still gets the same amount of pleasure. Now, this thrusting technique is a little complex so it might be hard to grasp the first time. If you're not 100% sure about how it works then you may want to read it through again, but once you get it, it can work wonders for you in the bedroom.

As men, in what way do we instinctively like to have sex? Generally, we men like to thrust hard and fast. It just comes naturally to us. And in porn, all the guys do it too. So it seems like the only sensible thing to do, right? Well, not exactly. Because what's the problem with thrusting hard and fast? Thrusting hard and fast causes way too much stimulation. And again, like you learned earlier, to last longer in bed you've got to reduce your overall stimulation to a controllable level.

Now, the funny thing is, in our desire to thrust hard and fast, we rarely take the time to think about what the woman likes. I mean, in porn women seem to be happy with hard and fast thrusting, but what about real life? Well, the truth is that in real life women generally like to be made love to compassionately and lovingly. This means that they don't need to be rammed super hard to experience an orgasm. When you take your time, enjoy foreplay, tease her a lot, build up lots of anticipation and very slowly and teasingly (two steps forward, one step back) start having sex with her, she will go crazy for you. You see, you've got to realize that women experience sex entirely differently from men.

Men are very much visual and like the look of hard and rough sex, whereas women like to feel things out and be appreciated. And in many other ways, we men experience sex very differently from women. So, when you take your time having sex and when you take things slow, you're speaking their language. They'll get into what you're doing and if you set things up right, she'll orgasm faster than you ever expected.

Many times you won't even have to be banging her 100mph to get her to orgasm. Sure, you can choose to increase the speed of your thrusting later on into sex, but you don't need to do it when starting. The bottom line of what I'm trying to get at is that taking things a little slower is okay. It's much more than okay, it's very much appreciated by women. And when you take things slow there are two very obvious benefits when it comes to meaning you last longer in bed...

Firstly, if you're going slower then you're giving yourself less stimulation, and as you know, with less stimulation you last longer. Secondly, if you start slowly, you're giving your penis more time to get used to being in the vagina. And the reason this is so important is that if you go in and start thrusting very fast then your body instinctively reacts with orgasm. However, if you go in very slowly then your penis has the chance to "acclimatize" or get used to the feeling of the vagina and therefore the initial powerful stimulating feeling that can trigger a very early orgasm goes away. The more time you spend in the vagina the less stimulated you will be by just being in there.

And once you've been thrusting very slowly for a minute or two, suddenly you can thrust faster and it's not a problem, whereas if you'd started thrusting fast at the beginning your body would have been overwhelmed with stimulation and not have lasted very long at all.

4. Control Your Hormones to Last Longer

In case you don't know what hormones are, they're chemicals released by the body into the bloodstream to influence the other parts of the body's processes. What happens during sex is that, depending on our emotions, different hormones get released into our bloodstream. And sometimes the hormones released into our bloodstream can encourage premature ejaculation. I'm talking about the hormones 'dopamine and adrenaline'. These two hormones are released when we experience emotions of fear, stress and over-excitement.

This means to last longer in bed, all you've got to do is find a few things you can do to stop yourself from experiencing these emotions before and during sex. Still, sound complicated? What this means is that you've got to figure out some ways to relax before and during sex. And one of the simplest ways to relax before and during sex (without doing anything too weird) is to use slow, deep breathing. Normally, when most men have sex, they tend to breathe very fast and shallow breaths. This has the effect of increasing tension in the body, creating fear, stress, and over-excitement. So, the simple cure to this is to just become aware of your shallow breathing and instead take in some very slow deep breaths.

As you take in these slow deep breaths, you'll begin to notice your body relaxing. You'll also observe your muscles becoming less tense. As you find your whole body relaxing your overall tension will drop. And like I said earlier, this reduction in fear, stress or overexcitement slows down the release of dopamine and adrenaline and therefore lasting longer comes naturally.

Try to keep sex at a relatively slow pace, at least in the beginning. Control your tempo if you can, and remember that sex isn't a race.

CHAPTER THREE

Erectile Dysfunction

In this chapter, we are going to discuss another very important health issue faced by a lot of men – erectile dysfunction.

Erectile dysfunction, or ED, is the inability to achieve or sustain an erection suitable for sexual intercourse. Causes include medications, chronic illnesses, poor blood flow to the penis, drinking too much alcohol, or being too tired.

Physical Causes of Erectile Dysfunction

Behind the scenes, a lot goes into achieving an erection. When you're turned on, nerves fire in your brain and travel down your spinal cord to your penis. There, muscles relax and blood flows into the blood vessels. The result, if all goes well, is a rigid penis, ready for sex. Unfortunately, all does not always go well. Many diseases - and, in some cases, their treatment - can lead to erectile dysfunction. So can injuries, lifestyle choices, and other physical factors. ED can often be treated, and finding the right cause can lead to successful treatment. The major causes of erectile dysfunction as stated below:

1. Diabetes: This chronic disease can damage the nerves and blood vessels that aid in getting an erection. When the disease has not been well controlled over time, it can double a man's risk of erection problems.

2. kidney disease: Kidney disease can affect many of the things you need for a healthy erection, including your hormones, blood flow to your penis, and parts of your nervous system. It can also sap your energy level and rob you of your sex drive. Drugs for kidney disease can also cause ED.

3. Neurological (nerve and brain) disorders: You can't get an erection without help from your nervous system, and diseases that disrupt signals between your brain and your penis can lead to ED. Such diseases include stroke, multiple sclerosis (MS), Alzheimer's disease, and Parkinson's disease.

4. Blood vessel diseases: Vascular diseases can block the blood vessels. That slows the flow of blood to the penis, making an erection difficult to get. Atherosclerosis (hardening of the arteries), high blood pressure, and high cholesterol are among the most common causes of ED.

5. Prostate cancer: Prostate cancer doesn't cause ED, but treatments can lead to temporary or permanent erectile dysfunction.

The physical causes of ED are not only disease-related. There are many other potential causes, including:

1. Surgery: Surgery for both prostate cancer and bladder cancer can damage nerves and tissues necessary for an erection. Sometimes the problem clears up, usually within 6 to 18 months. But the damage can also be permanent. If that happens, treatments exist to help restore your ability to have an erection.

2. Injury: Injuries to the pelvis, bladder, spinal cord, and penis that require surgery also can cause ED.

3. Hormone problems: Testosterone and other hormones fuel a man's sex drive, and an imbalance can throw off his interest in sex. Causes include pituitary gland tumours, kidney and liver disease, depression, and hormone treatment of prostate cancer.

4. Venous leak: To keep an erection, the blood that flows into your penis must stay in your penis. If it flows back out too quickly -- a condition called venous leak, in which the veins in your penis don't constrict properly -- you will lose your erection. Both injuries and disease can cause a venous leak.

5. Tobacco, alcohol, or drug use: All three can damage your blood vessels. That makes it difficult for blood to reach the penis, which is essential for an erection. If you have hardened arteries (arteriosclerosis), smoking will dramatically raise your risk of ED.

6. Prescription drugs: There are more than 200 prescription drugs that can cause ED.

7. Prostate enlargement: Prostate enlargement, a normal part of ageing for many men, may also play a role in ED.

ERECTION KILLERS

1. Depression

The brain is an often-overlooked erogenous zone. Sexual excitement starts in your head and works its way down. Depression can dampen your desire and can lead to erectile dysfunction. Ironically, many of the drugs used to treat depression can also suppress your sex drive and make it harder to get an erection, and they can cause a delay in your orgasm.

2. Alcohol

You might consider having a few drinks to get in the mood, but overindulging could make it harder for you to finish the act. Heavy alcohol use can interfere with erections, but the effects are usually temporary. The good news is that moderate drinking - one or two drinks a day -

might have health benefits like reducing heart disease risks. And those risks are like erectile dysfunction risks.

3. Medications

The contents of your medicine cabinet could affect your performance in the bedroom. A long list of common drugs can cause ED, including certain blood pressure drugs, pain medications, and antidepressants. Street drugs like amphetamines, cocaine, and marijuana can cause sexual problems in men, too.

4. Stress

It's not easy to get in the mood when you are overwhelmed by responsibilities at work and home. Stress can take its toll on many different parts of your body, including your penis. Deal with stress by making lifestyle changes that promote well-32 being and relaxation, such as exercising regularly, getting enough sleep, and seeking professional help when appropriate.

5. Anger

Anger can make the blood rush to your face, but not to the one place you need it when you want to have sex. It's not easy to feel romantic when you are raging, whether your anger is directed at your partner or not. Unexpressed anger or improperly expressed anger can contribute to performance problems in the bedroom.

6. Anxiety

Worrying that you won't be able to perform in bed can make it harder for you to do just that. Anxiety from other parts of your life can also spill over into the bedroom. All that worry can make you fear and avoid intimacy, which can spiral into a vicious cycle that puts a big strain on your sex life -- and relationship.

7. Middle-Aged Spread

Carrying extra pounds can impact your sexual performance, and not just by lowering your self-esteem. Obese men have lower levels of the male hormone testosterone, which is important for sexual desire and producing an erection. Being overweight is also linked to high blood pressure and the hardening of the arteries, which can reduce blood flow to the penis.

8. Self-Image

When you don't like what you see in the mirror, it's easy to assume your partner isn't going to like the view, either. A negative self-image can make you worry not only about how you look, but also about how well you are going to perform in bed. That performance anxiety can make you too anxious to even attempt sex.

9. Low Libido

Low libido isn't the same as erectile dysfunction, but a lot of the same factors that stifle an erection can also dampen your interest in sex. Low self-esteem, stress, anxiety, and certain medications can all reduce your sex drive. When all those worries are tied up with making love, your interest in sex can take a nosedive.

10. Your Health

Many different health conditions can affect the nerves, muscles, or blood flow that is needed to have an erection. Diabetes, high blood pressure, hardening of the arteries, spinal cord injuries, and multiple sclerosis can contribute to ED. Surgery to treat prostate or bladder problems can also affect the nerves and blood vessels that control an erection.

Exercise for Better Sexual Health

Exercise not only delivers some amazing health benefits - but it can also improve your sex life. Here's how.

1. Lower Risk of ED

The biggest boost exercise can give to your sex life is to lower your risk of erectile dysfunction. Exercise that helps open the arteries to benefit your heart will also increase blood flow to the penis.

One Harvard study of more than 31,000 men found that physically active men over age 50 were less likely to be impotent than inactive men. The exercisers had better erections, and those who were most active saw the most benefit. But even moderate levels of exercise, like a brisk 30-minute walk most days of the week, lowered the risk of ED. Other research suggests that many men with ED may even reverse their symptoms by getting fit.

Regular exercisers are also more likely than lazy people to have a healthy body weight - a key benefit, given that being overweight is another risk factor for ED.

2. Improved Symptoms of BPH

Physically active men may also have fewer symptoms of an enlarged prostate, a common condition called *benign prostatic hyperplasia* (BPH). Men with BPH often urinate frequently or have a weak stream. Men with more severe BPH symptoms may also have a low libido, trouble keeping an erection and enjoy sex less. A study published in the *Journal of Urology* found that active men cut their risk of urinary tract symptoms in half. There is no one best exercise for men with BPH. Getting 30 minutes of solid exercise on most days is enough to see benefits. And you can even break up your activity into 10-minute segments.

3. Better Semen Quality

If you want to have children, or think you might down the road, take note: A recent study in the *British Journal of Sports Medicine* suggests that men who worked out at a moderate to a vigorous intensity at least 15 hours a week had higher sperm counts than inactive men.

4. Fit for the Bedroom

When it comes to the strictly muscular aspect of sex, fit men have the advantage. Men in prime shape will find sex easier and less painful than men who don't exercise much, says Neal Pire, a fitness consultant to pro athletes. "If you don't exercise regularly, and especially if you never do crunches, you will feel soreness in your lower abdominals and your hip flexors after sex," he says. If you are partial to the missionary position, you might feel soreness in your chest muscles, he adds.

Exercise can help you feel more confident and energized both in and out of the bedroom, which can improve sex. When you feel good about yourself, and about how your partner sees you physically, you're going to be more relaxed and less distracted. Your best bet for overall enhanced sexual health is a well-rounded exercise regimen of strength, cardio, and flexibility training.

Exercise Regularly

Regular exercise can improve your health in many ways. Along with improving erectile function, exercise can:

- Strengthen the heart.
- Build energy levels.
- Lower blood pressure.
- Improve muscle tone and strength.
- Strengthen and build bones.
- Help reduce body fat.
- Help reduce stress, tension, anxiety, and depression.
- Boost self-image and self-esteem.
- Improve sleep.
- Make you feel more relaxed and rested.
- Make you look fit and healthy.

To get the most benefit, you should exercise at least 20 to 30 minutes, preferably on most days of the week. If you are a beginner, exercise for a few minutes each day and build up to 30 minutes. Discuss starting an exercise program with your doctor. When starting, you should plan a routine that is easy to follow and stick with. As the program becomes more routine, you can vary your exercise times and activities. Here are some tips to get you started.

How to Talk to Your Doctor about ED

Having trouble getting an erection can be embarrassing. No man wants to admit that he can't get it up. Some men are so embarrassed that they're even reluctant to talk to their doctor about erectile dysfunction. That's bad for several reasons. Erection difficulties can be an early warning sign of serious health problems, such as heart disease and diabetes. Erectile dysfunction can also be caused by certain medications, such as blood pressure drugs. And no matter what's causing your erection problems, your doctor can help, either with simple advice or medication.

Myths and Facts about Erectile Dysfunction

A subject like erectile dysfunction is bound to be surrounded with as much legend as fact when it comes to causes and treatments. Check out these common myths about ED and the facts to dispel the rumours.

Erectile Dysfunction and Age

Myth: ED is just a normal part of growing older and men just have to learn to live with it.

Fact: Although ED is more common among older men, that doesn't make it "normal" - or something you just have to live with. It's not unusual for older men to need more stimulation to help get them aroused than they did when they were younger. But there's no reason you should have to accept a lack of sexual function as one of the inevitable consequences of getting older. Many men can get erections and enjoy sex well into their senior years, and there's very likely no reason that you can't be one of them.

Myth: Erectile dysfunction doesn't hit younger men. It's only a problem for older guys.

Fact: Although erectile dysfunction is more common in men over 75, men of any age can develop erectile problems.

Erectile Dysfunction and Overall Health

Myth: ED may be upsetting, but there's nothing dangerous about it.

Fact: Although the ED itself isn't necessarily dangerous, ED is often one of the earliest warning signs of other underlying health conditions that can be quite serious. One of the most common underlying health conditions is diabetes. Erection problems can also be a symptom of heart problems such as hypertension (high blood pressure) or atherosclerosis, as well as hormone imbalances and neurological disorders such as Parkinson's disease. That's why it is essential to see your doctor if you have erectile dysfunction. Not only can a thorough medical examination help you identify the cause of the problem and find a treatment that can return you to a more active sex life, but it may also alert you to a bigger health condition that needs immediate treatment.

Myth: If you have trouble getting an erection, it's because you're not attracted to your partner.

Fact: There are many reasons why a man might experience erection problems. Although a lack of sexual attraction to one's partner might be one of them, it's far more likely to be something else.

CHAPTER FOUR

Aphrodisiac Foods You Must Eat

Did you know that certain foods are powerful aphrodisiacs? Here are some libido-lifting foods that will help improve your sex life.

The Indian Kamasutra states that before sex you should eat a meal of rice. The French King, Henry IV, drank a shot of cognac with egg yolk every morning to increase his "man powers". To increase potency, Italians ate chili peppers, chocolate, caviar, and oysters. These are just a few examples of how throughout history, there have been hundreds of foods and drinks that were believed to have special abilities for making men (and women) more "powerful" in bed.

Still to this day, men are always looking for natural ways to increase their potency. Sometimes, to enjoy sexual contact at its peak you have to restore the mental balance, get rid of the stress and produce some endorphins in the gym. However, you can also increase or awaken your desire, sexuality, sexual attraction, and sex drive by eating certain foods known as ***aphrodisiacs***.

From a scientific standpoint, many historically "powerful" aphrodisiacs may have had such strong results due to mere belief or their powers by users. While nowadays, because of science, many foods are helpful in your sex life because of the nutrients, vitamins, and minerals they contain. They improve your mental and physical health and can also help boost your testosterone levels.

Having a healthy body and mind will allow you to regain your lost interest in sex and strengthen your ability to perform. Here is a list of these natural aphrodisiacs for men, which will increase your sexual health and potency.

1. Almonds

This kind of nut has a great amount of vitamin B2, protein, vitamin E and calcium. Indians, Arabs, and Chinese have eaten almonds for centuries to increase their 38 sexual powers. Ayurveda, the traditional Indian medicine, even notes that almonds are a great food for brain activity and help to awaken sexual desire. Plus, Tim Ferris states in his book "The Four Hour Body" that he used almonds as a supercharger to boost his libido and sperm count around 4 hours before sex. This is a really good place to start when it comes to aphrodisiacs.

2. **Marzipan**

This almond paste is a common gourmet dessert which helps to increase sexual desire. As we spoke about above, almonds are a killer aphrodisiac and enjoying the paste as a dessert is a nice way to end the night with your lady. Almonds are grown in the East, Italy, Spain, and California – where they have the same reputation as a delicious, nutrient-dense food.

3. Honey

Also called the *food of the gods*, is a sweet elixir produced by bees from pollen. There are thousands of aromas of honey which all depend on the flowers from which the bees gathered nectar. All these scents are unique; from heavy, deep chestnut honey flavour to a light lavender and wild thyme smell. Alongside the aromas, honey is especially appreciated for its effects on one's sexual life. It is one of the best re-generators of sexual energy. Together with nuts, fruits, eggs and meat, it creates some of the best "turn-on" dishes. Avoid heated or filtered honey and instead opt for natural and raw honey, which has all the powers and aromas you need.

4. **Artichoke**

The mysterious hearts of artichokes are great aphrodisiacs, especially valued by the French. They believe that artichokes "warm up" the genitals. An artichoke stuffed with marinated shrimp is an extremely sensual dish, providing an unforgettable experience.

5. **Asparagus**

This is a time-tested drug for prostate diseases. Even its shape recalls the form of a phallus. It is also rich in asparagine – a widely known diuretic, which increases urinary activity. Since asparagus is rich in vitamin A, phosphorus, calcium, and potassium, it is officially classified as a booster of sexual desire. To get the most benefit, you should eat young shoots which are cut in spring. They have a mild taste; just do not cook them long.

6. **Avocado**

The name was given by the Aztecs, literally meaning testicles. This is due to the form of the fruit hanging on a tree resembling the male testicles. Other than looking like a man's set, avocado is a very nutritious fruit rich in protein, vitamin A, potassium, and non-essential fatty acids. These fatty acids will help your body produce testosterone, while the combination of all the nutrients provides a strong sexual boost. This sexual boost has been known and used for years.

7. **Banana**,

This is also a great booster of the male sex organ. Bananas are a great natural aphrodisiac and are rich in potassium and natural sugars. Indian traditional medicine classifies bananas as a "turn-on" food. A great recipe to spice them up a little bit is to take a bit of curry and butter and pour it over a banana. Sprinkle on some walnuts and you are good to go. Otherwise, you can just grab one for breakfast and it will give you a good sexual appetite throughout the day.

8. **Flower pollen**

It is more than just food. It has an incredible amount of nutrients including amino acids, vitamins, minerals, and superoxide dismutase, which has been shown to slow down ageing. While athletes from around the world use flower pollen to enhance strength and endurance, it is also shown to be one of the most effective passion-boosting products.

9. **Coconut**

Coconut has fantastic effects on the body. Indians say that coconuts increase the amount of sperm and cleanse the urinary bladder while eastern doctors recommend a coconut diet for tiring chronic diseases which take away all your energy. Combining coconut milk with honey is a nutritious drink, improving digestion and increasing sexual appetite. Another great breakfast/anytime recipe is pineapple juice, fresh papaya and grated fresh coconut mixed into a drink. It is rejuvenating and refreshing, refilling enzyme reserves, and stimulating sexual desire.

10. **Dates**,

They grow in Africa, Central Asia, and Southern California. Dates are the staple diet of many tropical and desert regions. According to Ayurveda, dates purify the blood and increase the amount of semen in men. The sugar from dates also gives enough energy for long, passionate sex. Because of this, dates are considered "sexual" food. An easy recipe is to take finely chopped, crushed dates, rolled in shredded coconut and fill them with blanched almonds. That's a triple-threat sexual booster.

11. **Eggs**,

This gift, full of protein, has been considered a sexual stimulant throughout the ages. So much so, that Casanova ate them before every love adventure. Scientifically this is because of the great boost in testosterone that is provided by the good cholesterol that eggs and butter provide. For a sensual dessert to get any woman in the mood, try some eggnog (egg mixed with milk, cream, honey, vanilla, and nutmeg). This, and starting your day off with a few eggs, is a surefire way to keep your sexual energy at its peak.

12. **Garlic**

Garlic helps to regulate the blood flow in your body, especially in your pelvic area. It is also widely used in Eastern and Indian medicine because of its natural antibiotic properties and is an irreplaceable tool in Italian cuisine (have you ever heard that Italians are very good lovers?). If you want to eat a bit of garlic before the night, the only thing you have to remember is to give a piece to your partner. Thus, both of you will have the same breath. In Eastern tradition, a good dish before the night is some garlic, fried in butter with eggs. You get the same benefits of eggs listed above plus a kick from the garlic.

13. **Mango**

If you could call any fruit "divine", it would be the mango. The Indian health book of Ayurveda describes it as an easily digestible, strength-giving and *arousing* fruit. This sensual fruit can be used as a dessert and shared between partners. The mango itself also looks like the testicles and this alone stimulates imagination and desire.

14. **Mushrooms**

Let's just say it. The cap of the mushroom looks like the head of the penis. This is enough to stimulate desire. But besides this, mushrooms are rich in zinc and it is believed that they are a great source of sexual energy.

15. **Okra**

Originally, African slaves brought okra to New Orleans, where the dishes with it became very popular. They believed that lady's fingers lit the fire of passion. While In Indian tradition, okra is recommended as a food that rejuvenates, energizes and turns on sexual desire.

16. **Olive oil**

It is the most nutritious and easily digestible oil of all vegetable oils. Since olive oil is rich in essential fatty acids, healthy sex organs are supplied with all the nutrients they need, while testosterone production is enhanced. In the morning, Greeks drink a sip of olive oil and eat a big spoon of raw honey (honey again, noticing a trend?) to cleanse the bile duct and strengthen the genitals. Natural olive oil is one of the most useful products out there.

17. Onion

There are different kinds of onions: red, white, yellow, brown, and Spanish. In Eastern tradition, onion is considered a diuretic, tonic, stimulant, cleaner of the blood and sexual booster. Onions are widely used in Eastern, Chinese, and European cuisine. In these cultures, it is believed that onion helps to keep up sexuality.

18. **Pistachios**

In central Asia and India, it is believed that pistachios arouse sexuality and cleanse the blood. Combine pistachios with honey and expect a nice, refreshed libido.

19. **Sesame seeds**

They are *very* nutritious and are widely used in the East. Sesame seeds are rich in vitamin E and this may be the reason they are called men's food. In India, it is believed that sesame seed prolongs life. If you want to increase your sexual activity, you should eat sesame oil with honey or halva; a sweet dish made of ground sesame and honey, which is worshipped as a sexual stimulant in the East.

20. **Wheat grass**

This is rich in vitamin E and is known as the sex vitamin. If you get it, buy wheatgrass in a vacuum pack, otherwise, in a day or two it will get a bitter taste.

21. **Parsley**

This is used around the world as a desire-enhancing food. Put some fresh herbs in salads or make juice and drink a couple of teaspoons three times per day to reap these powerful benefits.

22. **Mint and peppermint tea**

This provides the benefits of acting as an antiseptic, being anti-inflammatory, strengthening the heart, helping with insomnia, alleviating headaches, *and* acting as an aphrodisiac.

23. **Aloe**

Also known as the "plant of one hundred years," the juice from aloe leaves with a spoon of honey (one teaspoon three times per day) will activate your pelvic blood circulation and help you to perform sexually. You can buy liquid *aloe vera* extract from your local pharmacy and use it with natural and raw honey.

24. **Celery**

Celery is boring, bland, and only good for making wings look more appetizing. But celery *should* become your new best friend. Celery does amazing things for a man. It has been proven to increase your semen volume and provide a boost to your sexual potency through its high amounts of vitamin E, magnesium, potassium and zinc. It also contains arginine which increases blood flow to your genitals, resulting in stronger and longer erections.

25. Moringa Oleifera Seed and Leaf

It produces an androgenic effect by enhancing sexual drive through increased serum and testicular testosterone levels, increased blood flow to the male reproductive organs and stimulating the nervous system to enhance sexual desires (libido). Moringa seeds, when taken are reported to have a serious effect on the genitals. It makes the penis rise and increases the volume and thickens the sperm in men.

26. Grapefruit

Lycopene is one of those phytonutrients that is good for circulation and good for sexual issues. This Lycopene is found in grapefruit which is therefore one of the best fruits for erectile dysfunction/impotence.

27. Pineapple

It is also known as sex food for men. Pineapples are rich in Vitamin C which helps to increase the blood flow to the penis. This fruit for erectile dysfunction/ impotency contains magnesium which makes you feel energetic.

28. Watermelon

When you eat watermelon, it helps to alleviate erectile dysfunction. This seasonal fruit for erectile dysfunction contains amino acids called citrulline, which helps to relax and dilate the blood vessels much like Viagra!

29. Strawberry

It is nature's version of Viagra! Strawberry is one such fruit which will provide you with a lot of energy. Men who suffer from impotency should consume strawberries an hour before going to bed.

30. Goji Berries

It is an aphrodisiac fruit. Goji berry is one of the most powerful fruits for erectile dysfunction. It is a known fact that Goji berries offer a higher concentration of beta-carotene than most other fruits.

31. Kiwi

Kiwi has the best nutritional density. It is this fruit which has the amino acid arginine that helps in lowering blood pressure and increasing the blood flow to the penis. Therefore, it is one of the best fruits for impotency/erectile dysfunction.

Conclusion

As you can see, there are plenty of aphrodisiacs for you to take advantage of as a man. Cultures around the world have been doing it for centuries and now you can do it right from your kitchen. So, whether you're whipping up a nice dish for your lady friend or just trying to get your mojo flowing before a night out, these aphrodisiacs won't leave you hanging.

But most importantly, do not expect all aphrodisiacs to work like magic. The mentioned products can help you to improve your sexual life, and overall, they can improve your physical and mental health, but some effects may be very subtle. Some may be very pronounced. But the bottom line is a healthy body and soul means lots of *great* sex. So have fun.

Habits That May Cause Impotency in Men

Caffeine

If you are in the practice of drinking a lot of coffee or caffeinated drinks, then you better kick the habit. Higher levels of caffeine consumption are related to increased levels of impotence. So, chuck that morning coffee and switch to green tea.

Diet

Eating an unbalanced diet is a bad habit that is a sure way to cause impotency. The body needs all the essential nutrients for its proper functions. How can the body pump blood to the penis if it is not functioning properly? So, an unhealthy diet is a habit that causes erectile dysfunction.

Snoring

Snoring is a sign that your breathing is constantly disturbed during your sleep. Modern research has linked sleep apnea which causes snoring to impotency or erectly dysfunction. Those who snore during their sleep are twice as likely to suffer from impotence as those who do not.

Smoking

Smoking is a surefire way to reduce your blood circulation. Impotence has long been related to smoking or the regular use of tobacco. Quit the habit of smoking to improve blood circulation and prevent impotency.

Obesity

One of the most common causes of impotence is obesity. It is directly linked to erectile dysfunction. So, it is time to ditch those unhealthy food habits to combat your impotence. Start incorporating regular exercises like swimming, jogging or aerobics into your daily routine. They help you shed weight and improve blood circulation to your penis.

Sleep

If you do not catch up on the required 8 hours of sleep every day, your body will be fatigued and refuse to function properly. This will cause impotency.

Alcohol

Heavy alcohol use is a bad habit that causes impotency. Consumption of alcohol causes the blood vessels to constrict and hamper the free and easy movement of blood throughout the body. This unhealthy habit will obstruct the passage of blood to the penis and cause impotency.

Supplements

It is a common fact that even though we eat a lot, most of it is junk and we do not get the proper nutrition that we require. So, we try to make up for it by taking supplements. But taking supplements is a bad habit that causes impotency. If your body is not nourished properly, how can it sustain an erection?

9 798889 863533

Printed by Libri Plureos GmbH in Hamburg, Germany